Minds-In-Motion

The MAZE Handbook

For Teachers and Parents

by Candace S. Meyer, M.S.

MINDS-IN-MOTION FOR THE 21ST CENTURY STUDENT

There seems to be no debate that the current educational system in the United States is "broken" and that it needs to be inherently "fixed". Therefore, the focus is naturally drawn away from the child and towards the bureaucracy of the system. At Minds-In-Motion, our approach is different. We focus on building a better student, and on giving teachers proven tools they can use in their own classroom or whole school to create results.

The link between early physiological development and more complex cognitive abilities is one of the bedrock beliefs of Minds-In-Motion. In fact, we have built a company around research, which proves that spurring the physiological development of balance, in particular, in children leads to measurable gains academically, socially, behaviorally, and athletically. As educators and parents, we know that the ability to learn efficiently and effortlessly is one of the crucial foundations of success. A growing body of mainstream scientific research clearly points to the critical role that sensory/motor neural development through the vestibular system (balance/inner ear system) plays in the learning process. This all-important neural development cannot be bolstered by a traditional desktop learning approach. It requires addressing a whole host of physiological issues (detailed below) through integrating movements. These various exercises and protocols form the basis of the Minds-In-Motion MAZE, a simple, proven program that addresses the physiological needs of today's 21st Century learners.

How the Minds-In-Motion MAZE bolsters Components of Sensory/Motor Neural Development:

1. Our vestibular system acts as the CPU processor for our brain, and is responsible for coordinating and relaying vital information to our brain from the following sensory inputs:

- Inner ear
- Eyes
- Muscles and joints
- Jaw
- Fingertips and palms of hands
- Facial muscles
- Pressors on the soles of our feet
- Gravity receptors on our skin

2. Working as our sensory processor, the vestibular system also helps to regulate the following:

- Blood pressure
- Heart rate
- Breathing
- Digestion
- Elimination
- Speech ability
- Muscle tone
- Position of limbs
- Attention and arousal
- Immune system response

3. Scientific research validates that inefficiencies in the vestibular system can cause:

- Academic problems
- Speech problems
- Anxiety and stress
- Panic attacks
- Self-stimulating behaviors
- Poor muscle tone
- Bathroom issues
- Behavioral issues

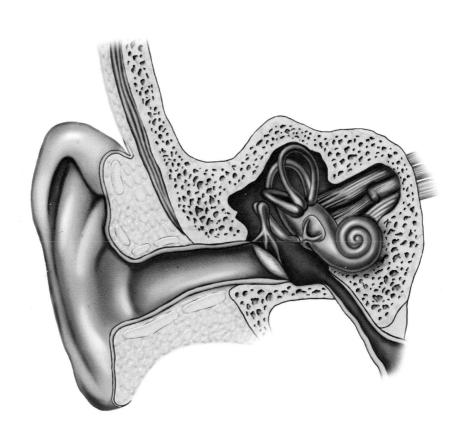

Step by Step Circuit to Success

The 15 daily Minds-In-Motion activities have been designed to develop and challenge a student's balance and learning capabilities. The entire circuit takes only three to five minutes to complete! It needs very little space to implement, and very few monitors to supervise it. Many schools set up the maze in vacant classrooms, meeting rooms or hallways. Some schools run the entire student population through in a staggered fashion first thing in the morning. Other schools assign classes at specific times to visit the Maze each day. Each school's needs are different; however, a Maze can be designed to work at any school or at any home. See examples of Minds-In-Motion designs in back of book.

The Minds-In-Motion Maze boasts a wide range of simple methods to:
- alleviate clumsiness and disorganization
- improve vision skills for reading
- improve handwriting skills
- increase tracking of digits in math
- combat double vision
- empower self control
- increase focusing ability
- improve tonal quality of speech
- improve eye-hand coordination
- and affect many more sensory and motor integration issues

ON THE FOLLOWING PAGES, each basic motor activity of the Maze is outlined in detail, explaining how to properly perform each activity, why the activity is educationally and physiologically important and how the activity translates to classroom skills. Also included in this book is a compilation of activities to update the Maze weekly. It is important to keep it fresh and challenging for a whole school year. Each skill builds upon the previous one to speed along sensory integration and motor development to the fullest.

Equipment lists

BALANCE BEAMS
- Use at least 2 boards of varying thickness
- 1"x4"x12' (or whatever length your space can accommodate)
- 2"x4"x12'
- 4"x4"x12'
- 3"x4"x12' (you can use duct tape to tape a 1x4 and 2x4 together if a 3x4 board is hard to attain)

BEAN BAGS (5-6 DOZEN)
- Use varying sizes and weights
- Vary the contents between sand, beans, rice, popcorn or gravel

BALANCE BOARDS (5-6 INDIVIDUAL BOARDS)
- App. 12"x22" each
- A variety of balance boards work well: wooden, hard plastic, wobble boards, adjustable rockers

EYE TRACKING PENCILS/WANDS (4-6 PENCILS)
- Pencil toppers can change by the season (apples, ghosts, santa, Easter eggs, etc.)

ITEMS FOR CLIMBING OVER
- Wooden steps or varying heights
- Cardboard building blocks
- Cones and cross-bars, etc.

PADS TO STOMP ON
- Carpet Squares
- Foam interlocking squares
- Cushioned floor tiles that stick on the floor

TUMBLING MATS
- 2 (4'x8') mats hooked together work well

VISION BEAD STRINGS
- (8-9 strings mounted on a 1"x2"x8')

MISCELLANEOUS
- containers to keep beanbags, pencils, etc.

Minds-In-Motion

MAZE

15 Developmental Steps
for Brain/Body Integration

Strong Arm Push

QUICK TIP
Push straight out from the chest perpendicular to the wall.

How? Students stand facing a wall, then push against the wall with the palms of their hands. Encourage pushing with as much force as possible for a count of ten.

Why? Pushing activates pressors in palms of hands which are rich in vestibular connections. It also stimulates proprioceptive (muscle and joint) development in hands and arms.

Benefit? Pushing develops fine motor control in handwriting. It also develops the ability to focus eyes on a sentence on the chalkboard as one continues to copy words on paper while seated at a desk.

"Over 80% of the nervous system is involved in processing or organizing sensory input, thus the brain is primarily a sensory processing machine." –Carol Stock Kranowitz, M.A., 1998

Bean Bag Boogie

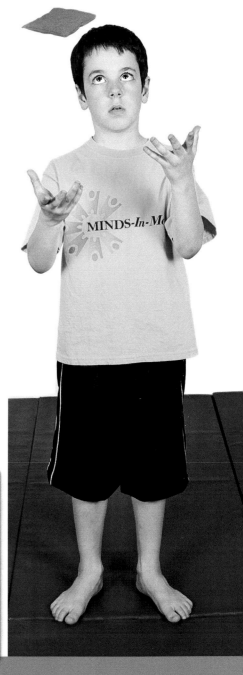

How? While walking along a given path, students throw and catch a beanbag in various designated patterns. Students are encouraged to always follow the bag with their eyes. Starting with a 2-hand catch, students will progress through several skill levels of tossing and catching as the year ensues.

Why? Following an object with the eyes develops eye-hand coordination, focusing, and eye tracking.

Benefit? Bean Bag Boogie develops fine motor control, while helping coordinate eyes and hands (visual-motor control) for writing, board-to-seat work, and computer work.

QUICK TIP
Eyes must focus on the beanbag at all times.

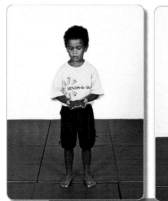
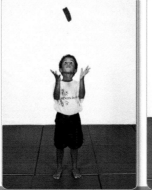
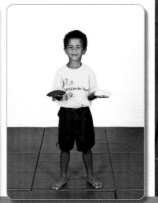

"Sensory motor integration is fundamental to school readiness." *–Housten, 1982; Hannaford, 1995*

Eye to Eye

QUICK TIP
Student's head should NOT move, only the eyes.

How? Instructor stands in front of student and moves pencil (with bright topper or eraser) in front of student's eyes (app. 14 inches away) while student follows the object with his/her eyes. Instructor moves the pencil in the following pattern:

2 horizontal - 2 vertical - 2 circles clockwise

2 circles counterclockwise - 2 horizontal

2 convergence training (going in toward the nose)

Why? Eye exercises strengthen eye muscles for eye tracking and eye-teaming (coordinated movement of eyes).

Benefit? Increased ocular control provides fluidity in reading and tracking of digits in math.

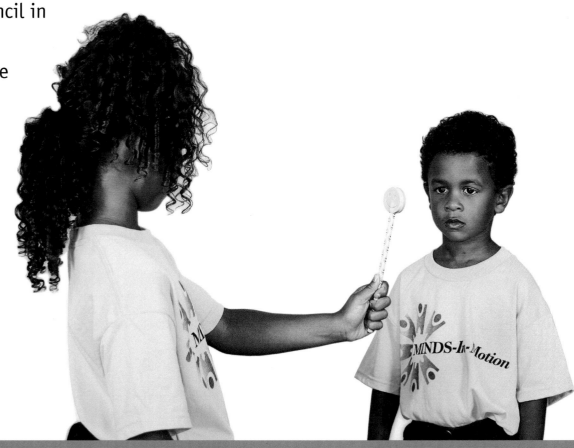

"There is a rapidly growing awareness that children who do not learn to read efficiently are children who have not developed good functional visual skills" *–Dr. James Kimple, 1997*

Jelly Roll

How? Students roll on a mat on the floor in a predetermined manner.

Why? Rolling provides vestibular stimulation to the brain and builds core strength.

Benefit? Students increase the ability to know where they are in 'space and time' while developing the spatial orientation of an object or a line of print.

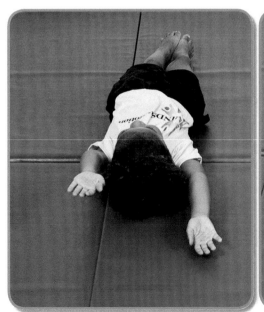 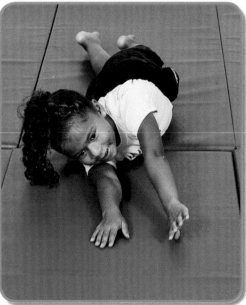 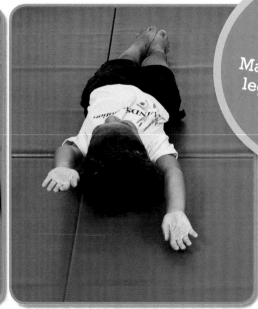

QUICK TIP
Make sure his/her legs are straight.

"When messages come in, and motor messages go out, in a synchronized way, our bodies can do what we need to do in an organized way." *–Carol Stock Kranowitz, M.A., 1998*

Puppy Dog Crawl

How? Students crawl on hands and knees down on the floor in a given direction for a specified distance.

Why? Crawling develops cross-lateral hand and leg coordination, increases convergence of eyes, and establishes timing in the brain.

Benefit? Thoughts are more organized when both hemispheres of the brain are cross integrated.

QUICK TIP
Eyes should be following the lead of the hands.

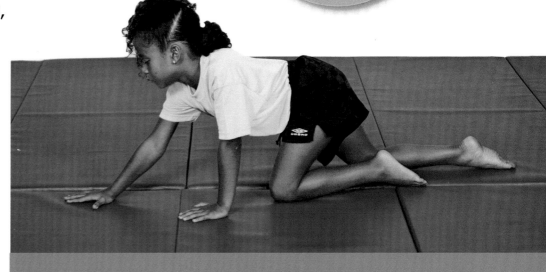

"Laterality is the internal awareness of "sidedness". A basic component of the development of laterality is proper, sufficient crawling. *—Dr's. Odell & Cook, 1997*

Climb Every Mountain

QUICK TIP
Feet should go up and over each obstacle rather than around the side.

How? Students step over hurdles or obstacles of varying heights.

Why? Stepping over objects develops depth perception while increasing eye-foot coordination and balance.

Benefit? Eyes focus better on a page of print due to increased binocularity of eyes (depth perception).

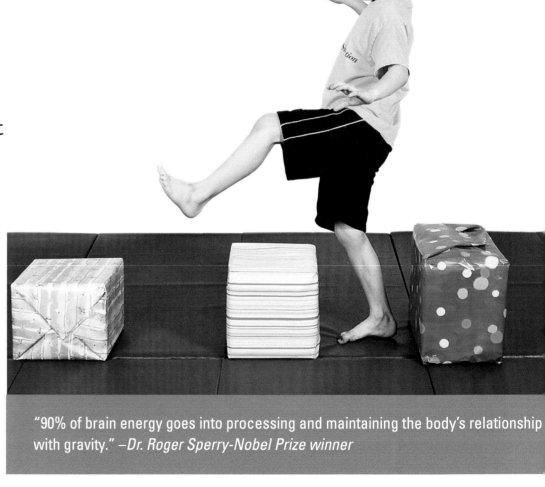

"90% of brain energy goes into processing and maintaining the body's relationship with gravity." –Dr. Roger Sperry-Nobel Prize winner

Monster Mash

QUICK TIP
Encourage students to stomp really hard on pads.

How? Students stomp down hard on padded shapes or blocks laid out on floor in patterns.

Why? Stomping provides somatosensory stimulation through the feet and legs to the brain while increasing the sense of balance. Pressors on the soles of the feet are rich in neural connections to the vestibular system.

Benefit? This exercise enables students to walk, stand, and sit in a controlled manner.

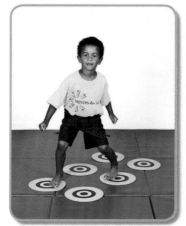
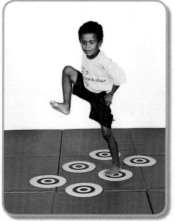
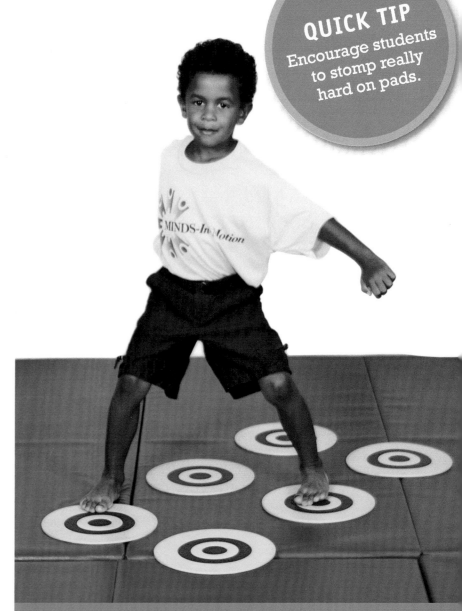

The Minds-In-Motion MAZE Handbook

"Whether we are aware of it or not, vestibular processing is involved in everything we do. Without our vestibular system, we could not stay upright, could not sit, stand or run!."
—Nancy Sokol Green, 2003

Eye Can Converge

QUICK TIP
Don't let them favor one eye or the other! Keep head perpendicular to string.

How? Students hold a Beaded String (3 beads affixed to a 5 foot string) in their hand and focus on each differently colored bead one at a time while counting to 10 for each bead.

Why? This eye exercise helps develop eye-convergence or eye-binocularity.

Benefit? Convergence practice aids students in focusing upon letters and numbers with no double vision to create a strong SINGLE (fused) vision.

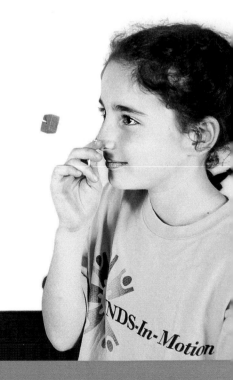

"70% of the children who have specific reading problems have been found to have problems in their visual syste that relate to movements of the eyes, depth perception, and finding targets (fixation)." *–Dr. Billye Ann Cheatum, 2*

Jumping Jack Flash

QUICK TIP
Students should land on both feet together at the same time.

How? Students do a standing "broad jump" between two (or more) designated lines drawn or taped to the floor.

Why? Jumping Jack Flash develops eye-foot coordination and sense of balance while fine-tuning reaction times through improved motor planning.

Benefit? This exercise perfects students' reaction times in problem solving, response time in general, and in judging distances.

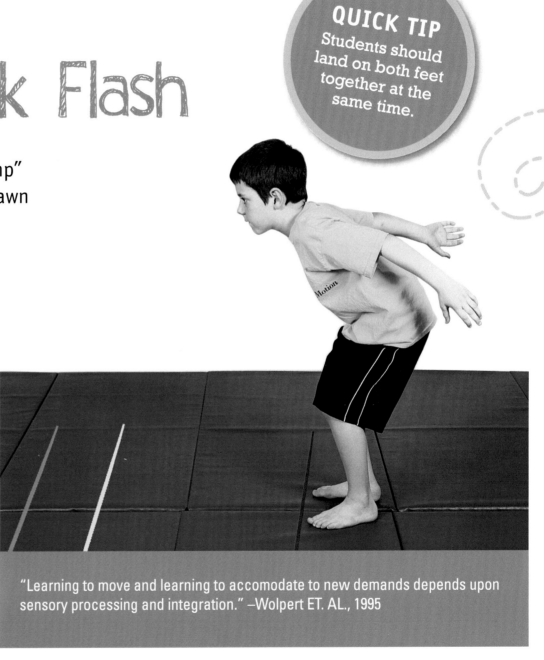

"Learning to move and learning to accomodate to new demands depends upon sensory processing and integration." –Wolpert ET. AL., 1995

Cross Walk

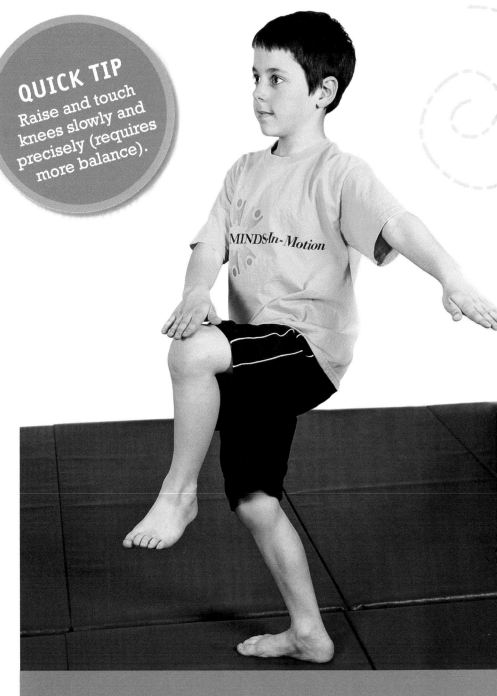

QUICK TIP
Raise and touch knees slowly and precisely (requires more balance).

How? Students slowly walk a given distance lifting knees high while touching alternating knees with opposite hands.

Why? Crossing the midline of the body is critical for developing the bilateral coordination of the body.

Benefit? Cross Walk helps develop laterality (sidedness) in students by building the corpus callosum (connecting neural pathways between the two hemispheres of the brain) which speeds up brain processing.

"Children experience movement with joy. They learn most when there is j[o] in learning." —*Kiphard, 2000*

Balance Board Bash

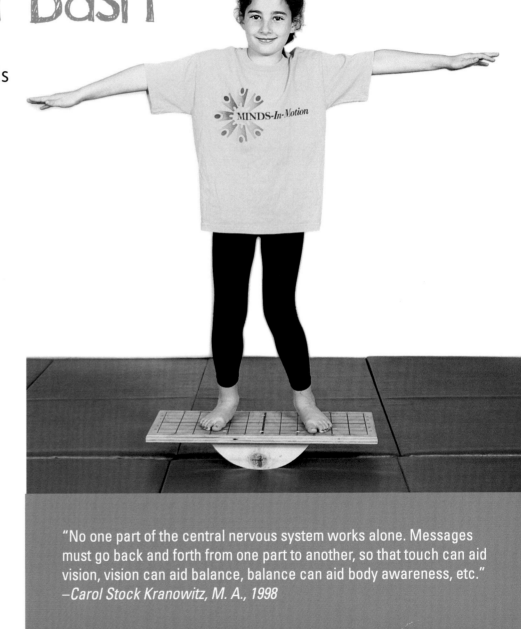

How? Students stand on wooden balance boards training their bodies to suspend in balance.

Why? Balancing stimulates visual and auditory processing.

Benefit? Balance Board Bash is key in ensuring students' proprioceptive, visual, and vestibular systems are intact to allow for maximum mental processing.

QUICK TIP
Make sure the feet are placed equal distance from center of the board.

"No one part of the central nervous system works alone. Messages must go back and forth from one part to another, so that touch can aid vision, vision can aid balance, balance can aid body awareness, etc."
–Carol Stock Kranowitz, M. A., 1998

The Beam Team

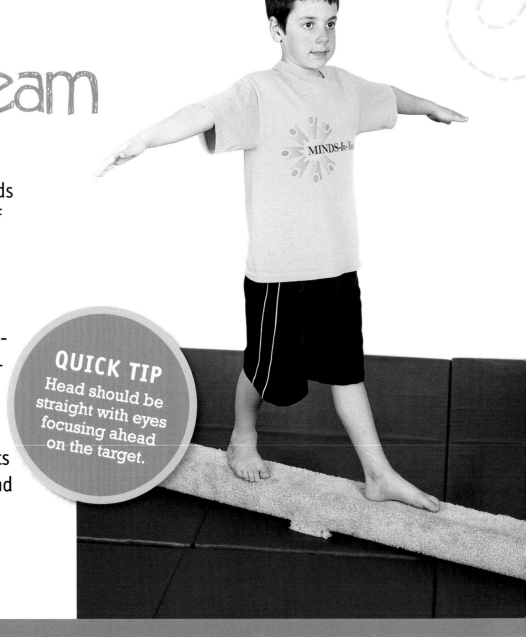

How? Students walk on long wooden boards (1"x4"x12ft.) or (2"x4"x12ft.) in a variety of manners to develop balance.

Why? By following a regimen of balancing exercises of increasing difficulty, students develop balance, fluid motor control, and maximize brain recalibration.

Benefit? Balance development in students alleviates clumsiness and disorganization, and improves visual-motor control, such as:

- spacing letters and numbers on a line
- size constancy of letters
- staying between two lines on paper

QUICK TIP
Head should be straight with eyes focusing ahead on the target.

"Proper neural pathways are laid with children aquire sensory motor skills through play and specific movements. " —Miller & Melamed, 1989

The Electric Slide

How? Students side-step along a designated "path" keeping their eyes, face, feet and whole body parallel to the wall. Move sideways by taking a step to the side, then sliding the following foot along until it touches the lead foot. Halfway through the path, students should turn 180 degrees and continue on, leading with the other leg.

Why? The Electric Slide develops laterality, directionality, and spatial awareness in the brain/body in an integrative whole-body movement.

Benefit? This activity enhances bilateral integration in the brain, which will allow students to organize their 'space and time' more efficiently.

QUICK TIP
Have students position their faces as close to the wall as possible without touching the wall.

"Directionality is the external, or "out of space" awareness of 'sidedness.' A good sense of directionality helps a child recognize quickly, without having to figure it out, the difference between b and d, was and saw, and which is right and which is left." –Dr's Odell & Cook, 1997

Step Back

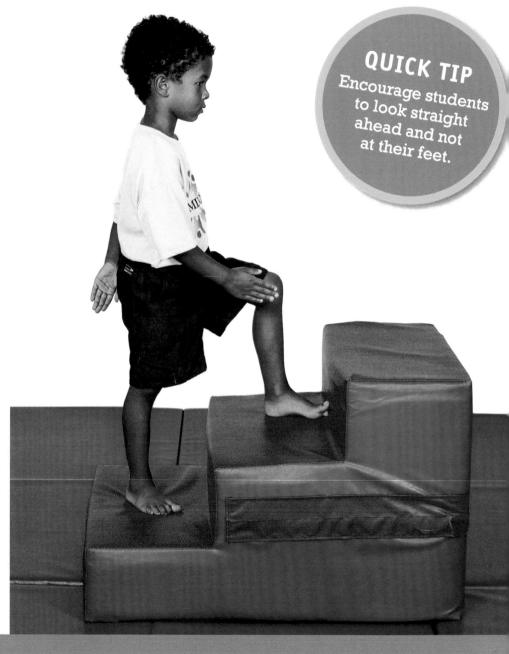

QUICK TIP
Encourage students to look straight ahead and not at their feet.

How? Students walk "backward" up or down a set of stairs holding onto a rail for support.

Why? Walking stairs backward develops whole body coordination moving in a posterior plane, and further enhances motor planning and depth perception.

Benefit? Step Back increases motor planning and learning how to do things without looking:

- For example, buttoning coat without looking, walking backwards without looking, etc.

"Without our vestibular system, we could not differentiate between moving in a circle versus moving in a straight line. We could not keep our eyes steady on a target even when our bodies are in motion."
—*Nancy Sokol Green, 2003*

Skip to My Lou

How? Students skip down a designated "lane" while swinging their arms cross laterally in an exaggerated fashion.

Why? Skipping develops bi-lateral integration of brain hemispheres while improving rhythmic motor development in a smooth coordinated manner.

Benefit? This exercise enhances motor planning in students, increasing their learning capabilities and developing essential automaticity of the brain/body. If a child has to think through a task first instead of performing it automatically, extra energy is expended to accomplish each task.

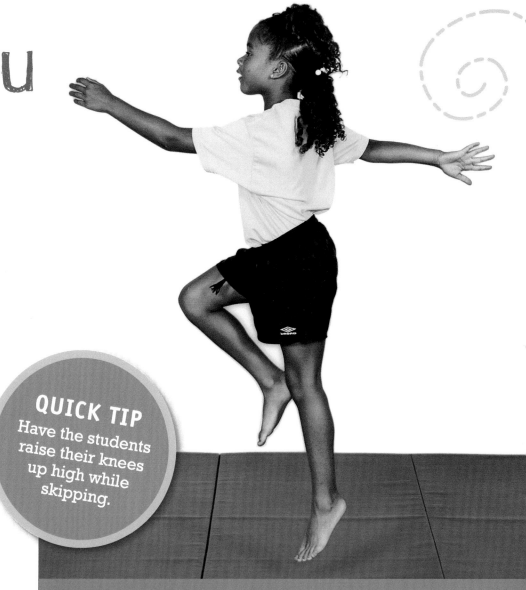

QUICK TIP
Have the students raise their knees up high while skipping.

"A child who is still in the laterality stage (does not know right from left) or lacks directionality (has not gained a sense of up/down, before/behind) will continue to get letters like b, d, p, q mixed up."
– *Dr. Billye Ann Cheatum, 2000*

Extra TIPS for a Successful Maze

MOST IMPORTANT: Remember to encourage [not reprimand]. An occasional "Oh, my, look at Billy...now that's the way to do it right!"; "You did it, Tiffany! Look how far you jumped!" will solve a lot of problems proactively!

1. STRONG ARM PUSH

- Good skill to place before Eye to Eye or Eye Can Converge (as both of these take more time to do).
- Arms should shake because the student is pushing so hard.

2. BEAN BAG BOOGIE

- Encourage students to visualize what ingredients are in their beanbags each time they toss them, but don't divulge the ingredients! Could be corn, rice, beans, sand, gravel, etc.
- Students should not throw beanbag higher than their head [unless specified in the skill].

3. EYE TO EYE

- The tracking pencil should be held app. 12 -14 inches in front of the student's eyes.
- For younger students, a larger item (such as a small stuffed animal) may be used.

- Vary the patterns of movement to ensure the student is truly following the tracking pencil.

4. JELLY ROLL

- Encourage the students to keep their arms straight down to the side for the basic roll.
- Encourage students to maneuver their bodies to stay on the mat rather than stopping and scooting back up on mat.

5. PUPPY DOG CRAWL

- Students should stare at the lead hand in the front as they crawl. [So they are moving their head back and forth focusing on right hand, then left, right, then left, etc.
- When army crawling, make sure students' legs and arms move cross-laterally.

6. CLIMB EVERY MOUNTAIN

- Change "mountain" often.
- Cones with rods placed at varying levels can be used effectively for students to climb over or under.

7. MONSTER MASH

- Reconfigure the pattern of the pads often.
- Taped "X"s on floor may be used in place of pads.
- The higher the students raise their legs the more balance it requires.

8. EYE CAN CONVERGE

- (Alternative method) Line up all 8-9 students on strings before starting. Call out 1st, 3rd, 2nd, 3rd, etc. bead in a random pattern for students to focus upon.
- Make sure children are holding beaded string perpendicular to nose, between thumb and bent finger, with thumb touching nose.
- Hold string tight.
- Students should see 2 strings (which is an optical illusion).

9. JUMPING JACK FLASH

- Legs should be bent together and should stay together as they jump.
- Arms should be bent and rotate back, then forwards to pump momentum into their jump.

10. CROSS WALK

- Encourage students to lift knees up high.
- Always touch the opposite side of body to make those neural connections.

11. BALANCE BOARD BASH

- Sandpaper "X"s glued onto the boards equidistance from center are helpful for placing feet correctly.
- Students should look straight ahead and not down at their feet.
- Students should try to stay balanced, not moving up and down constantly [younger students may have to keep moving at first, until they learn to balance].

12. THE BEAM TEAM

- Encourage students to go slowly and put their heel in front each time so it touches their toes. Heel – toe – heel – toe.
- Place a visual target "X" on the wall in front of and on the wall behind the students at eye level.

13. MUSIC

- Play calming, soothing music while students are going through maze if possible.
- On Fridays, pick up the tempo by playing Walt Disney favorites, popular songs, etc. to liven up the atmosphere!

Minds-In-Motion

MAZE

Sample diagrams

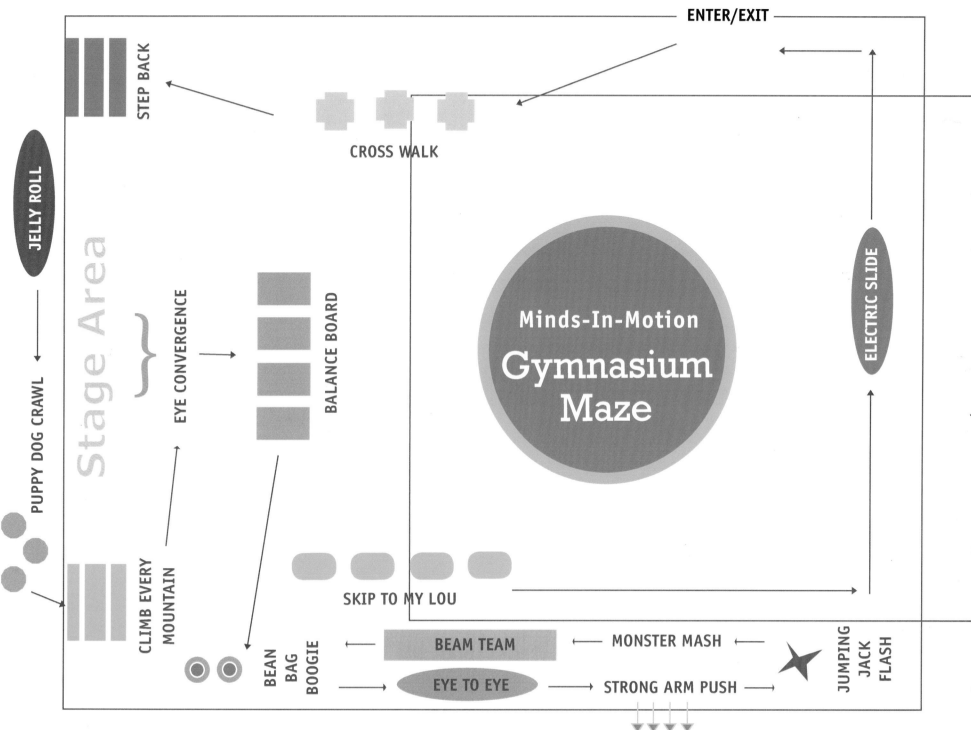

ENTER/EXIT

STEP BACK

JELLY ROLL

PUPPY DOG CRAWL

Stage Area

EYE CONVERGENCE

BALANCE BOARD

CROSS WALK

Minds-In-Motion
Gymnasium Maze

ELECTRIC SLIDE

CLIMB EVERY MOUNTAIN

BEAN BAG BOOGIE

SKIP TO MY LOU

BEAM TEAM

MONSTER MASH

EYE TO EYE

STRONG ARM PUSH

JUMPING JACK FLASH

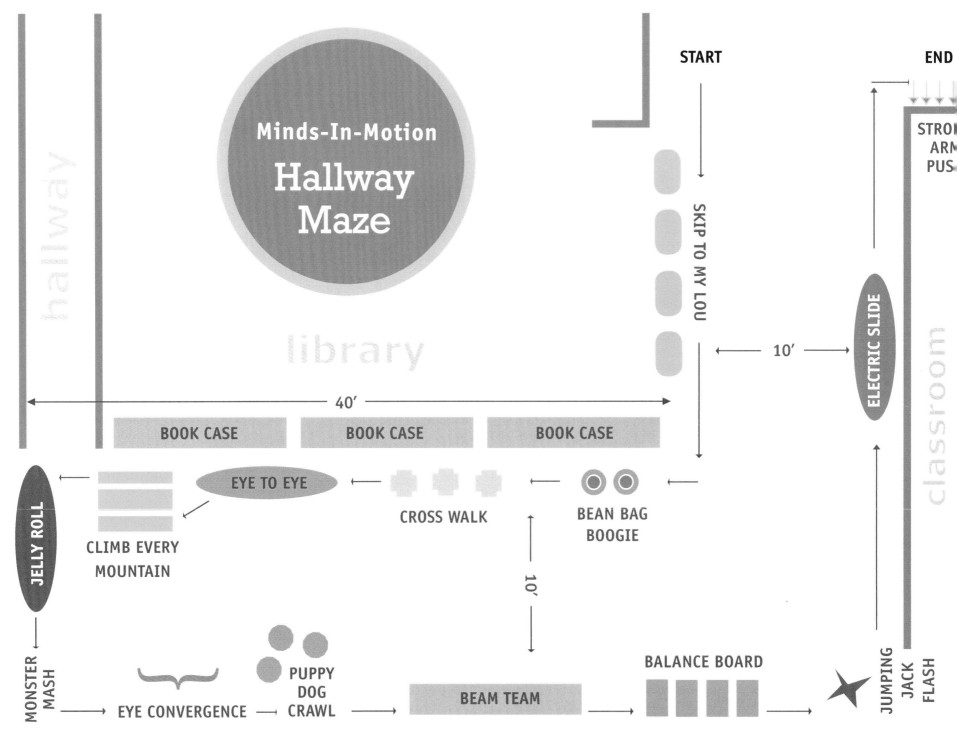

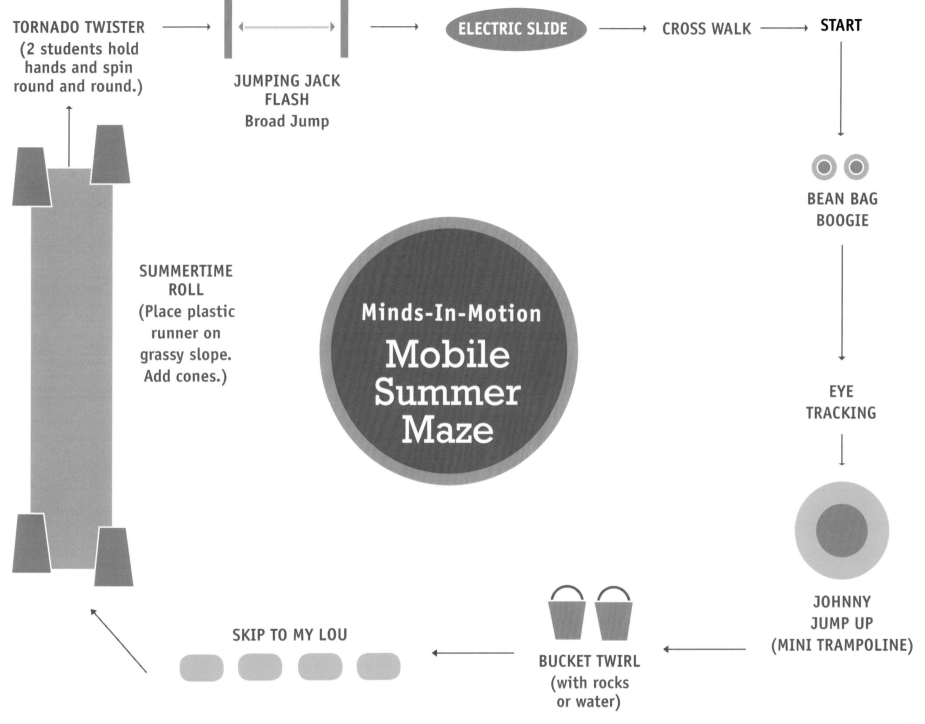

TORNADO TWISTER
(2 students hold hands and spin round and round.)

JUMPING JACK FLASH
Broad Jump

ELECTRIC SLIDE → CROSS WALK → **START**

BEAN BAG BOOGIE

SUMMERTIME ROLL
(Place plastic runner on grassy slope. Add cones.)

Minds-In-Motion
Mobile Summer Maze

EYE TRACKING

JOHNNY JUMP UP
(MINI TRAMPOLINE)

BUCKET TWIRL
(with rocks or water)

SKIP TO MY LOU

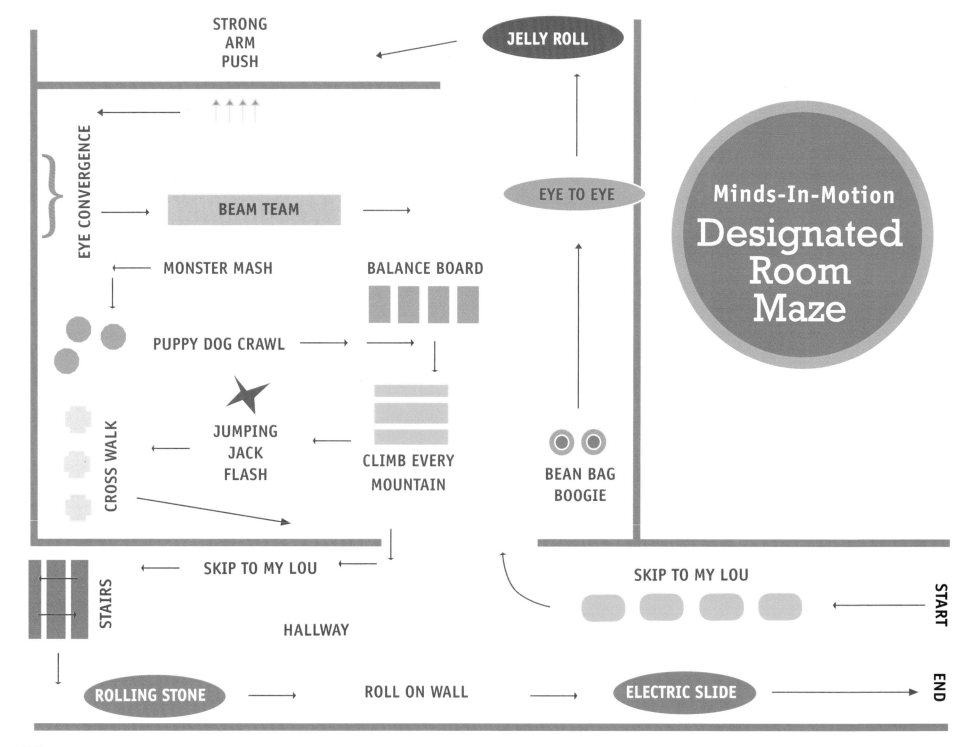

STRONG ARM PUSH

JELLY ROLL

EYE CONVERGENCE

EYE TO EYE

Minds-In-Motion
Designated Room Maze

BEAM TEAM

MONSTER MASH

BALANCE BOARD

PUPPY DOG CRAWL

CROSS WALK

JUMPING JACK FLASH

CLIMB EVERY MOUNTAIN

BEAN BAG BOOGIE

STAIRS

SKIP TO MY LOU

SKIP TO MY LOU

START

HALLWAY

ROLLING STONE

ROLL ON WALL

ELECTRIC SLIDE

END

Minds-In-Motion
MAZE

36 weekly routines

Minds-In-Motion **WEEK 1**

Each week changes will be made to some of the stations, increasing the skill level and intensity. If no change is designated, just continue with the basic movement as indicated on week 1:

1. SKIP TO MY LOU	Skip along designated "path" with your arms swinging cross-laterally while pumping your arms.
2. ELECTRIC SLIDE	Side-step along a designated wall keeping your eyes, face, feet and whole body facing forward, but moving sideways by taking a step to the side, then sliding the following foot along until it touches the lead foot. Halfway through the path, you should turn 180 degrees and continue on, leading with the other foot. You should get as close to the wall as possible without touching it.
3. BEAN BAG BOOGIE	Throw and catch a bean bag starting with a 2-hand catch and always following the bag with your eyes, while always moving along the circuit. You will progress through several skill levels of throwing and catching as the year ensues.
4. EYE TO EYE	Instructor stands in front of student and moves pencil slowly (with bright topper or eraser) in front of student's eyes (app. 14 inches away) while student follows the object with his/her eyes. Instructor moves the pencil in the following pattern: 2 horizontal - 2 vertical - 2 circles clockwise - 2 circles counterclockwise - 2 moving in towards nose
5. JUMPING JACK FLASH	Do a standing "broad jump" between two designated lines drawn or taped to the floor.
6. JELLY ROLL	Roll on a mat on the floor in a predetermined manner.
7. CROSS WALK	Slowly walk a given distance lifting knees high while touching alternating knee with opposite hand while other arms is held out to side.
8. BALANCE BOARD BASH	Stand on wooden balance boards training your body to suspend in balance.
9. CLIMB EVERY MOUNTAIN	Step over hurdles or obstacles of varying heights.
10. BEAM TEAM	Walk on long wooden boards in a variety of manners to develop balance. Always turn around at midpoint; continue by walking backwards.
11. MONSTER MASH	Stomp down hard on padded shapes or blocks laid out on floor in pattern.
12. PUPPY DOG CRAWL	Crawl on hands and knees down on the floor in a given direction for a specified distance.
13. EYE CAN CONVERGE	Hold "Eye Beads" (3 beads affixed to a 4 foot string) in your hand and focus on each differently colored bead one at a time while counting to 10 for each bead. For younger students, have them say color of bead, instead of counting.
14. STRONG ARM PUSH	Stand facing a wall, then push against the wall with the palms of your hands. Try pushing with as much force as possible for a count of ten.
15. STEP BACK	Walk "backwards" up a set of stairs holding onto a rail for support.

Minds-In-Motion WEEK 2

Each week changes will be made to some of the stations, increasing the skill level and intensity. If no change is designated, just continue with the basic movement as indicated on week 1:

1. SKIP TO MY LOU	
2. ELECTRIC SLIDE	
3. BEAN BAG BOOGIE	Throw a beanbag up in the air and try to touch it (NOT kick it) with your **RIGHT** foot when it comes down. Do this 10 times, while moving along the circuit.
4. EYE TO EYE	
5. JUMPING JACK FLASH	
6. JELLY ROLL	
7. CROSS WALK	
8. BALANCE BOARD BASH	
9. CLIMB EVERY MOUNTAIN	
10. BEAM TEAM	Holding your arms straight out to each side, walk down the beam turning backward at midpoint, while keeping your eyes on the fixation point. (Black X on wall)
11. MONSTER MASH	
12. PUPPY DOG CRAWL	
13. EYE CAN CONVERGE	
14. STRONG ARM PUSH	
15. STEP BACK	

Minds-In-Motion **WEEK 3**

Each week changes will be made to some of the stations, increasing the skill level and intensity. If no change is designated, just continue with the basic movement as indicated on week 1:

1. SKIP TO MY LOU	
2. ELECTRIC SLIDE	
3. BEAN BAG BOOGIE	Throw a beanbag up in the air and try to touch it (NOT kick it) with your **LEFT** foot when it comes down. Do this 10 times, while always moving along the circuit.
4. EYE TO EYE	
5. JUMPING JACK FLASH	
6. JELLY ROLL	Roll with your head at opposite side of mat from last week.
7. CROSS WALK	
8. BALANCE BOARD BASH	
9. CLIMB EVERY MOUNTAIN	
10. BEAM TEAM	Holding your **LEFT** arm extended out level with your shoulder, walk down the beam.
11. MONSTER MASH	
12. PUPPY DOG CRAWL	
13. EYE CAN CONVERGE	
14. STRONG ARM PUSH	
15. STEP BACK	

Minds-In-Motion WEEK 4

Each week changes will be made to some of the stations, increasing the skill level and intensity. If no change is designated, just continue with the basic movement as indicated on week 1:

1. SKIP TO MY LOU	
2. ELECTRIC SLIDE	
3. BEAN BAG BOOGIE	Throw a beanbag up in the air. Say "right", or "left" or say "both". Then catch with your right hand, the left hand, or both hands. Follow your command!
4. EYE TO EYE	
5. JUMPING JACK FLASH	
6. JELLY ROLL	Roll with your head at opposite side of mat from last week.
7. CROSS WALK	
8. BALANCE BOARD BASH	
9. CLIMB EVERY MOUNTAIN	
10. BEAM TEAM	Holding your **RIGHT** arm extended out level with your shoulder, walk down the beam.
11. MONSTER MASH	
12. PUPPY DOG CRAWL	
13. EYE CAN CONVERGE	
14. STRONG ARM PUSH	Push wall with **RIGHT** hip.
15. STEP BACK	

Minds-In-Motion **WEEK 5**

Each week changes will be made to some of the stations, increasing the skill level and intensity. If no change is designated, just continue with the basic movement as indicated on week 1:

1. SKIP TO MY LOU	
2. ELECTRIC SLIDE	
3. BEAN BAG BOOGIE	Throw a bean bag up in the air. When it reaches the top of its trajectory, close your eyes and try to catch it with your eyes closed. Repeat 10 times.
4. EYE TO EYE	
5. JUMPING JACK FLASH	
6. JELLY ROLL	
7. CROSS WALK	Take turns touching each elbow to the opposite knee as you cross walk.
8. BALANCE BOARD BASH	
9. CLIMB EVERY MOUNTAIN	
10. BEAM TEAM	Hold both arms out to the side of your body, level with your shoulders. Hold your palms up while walking on beam.
11. MONSTER MASH	
12. PUPPY DOG CRAWL	
13. EYE CAN CONVERGE	
14. STRONG ARM PUSH	Push wall with **RIGHT** hip.
15. STEP BACK	Walk "backwards" up a set of stairs holding onto a rail for support.

Minds-In-Motion WEEK 6

Each week changes will be made to some of the stations, increasing the skill level and intensity. If no change is designated, just continue with the basic movement as indicated on week 1:

1. SKIP TO MY LOU	
2. ELECTRIC SLIDE	While sliding, clap high twice above your head, then clap twice low behind your back.
3. BEAN BAG BOOGIE	Take 2 bean bags and throw them in rhythmic sequence. For example: Left hand - 2 times; right hand - 1 time. Continue at least 10 times.
4. EYE TO EYE	
5. JUMPING JACK FLASH	
6. JELLY ROLL	
7. CROSS WALK	
8. BALANCE BOARD BASH	While balancing, clap high twice above your head, then clap twice low behind your back, keep repeating while you count to 10.
9. CLIMB EVERY MOUNTAIN	New items to climb over! [Reconfigure your hurdles or get new items for the students to step over.]
10. BEAM TEAM	Hold your arms out in front of you. Hold your palms down while walking forward on the beams. (like Frankenstein!)
11. MONSTER MASH	
12. PUPPY DOG CRAWL	
13. EYE CAN CONVERGE	
14. STRONG ARM PUSH	
15. STEP BACK	

Minds-In-Motion WEEK 7

Each week changes will be made to some of the stations, increasing the skill level and intensity. If no change is designated, just continue with the basic movement as indicated on week 1:

1. SKIP TO MY LOU	
2. ELECTRIC SLIDE	
3. BEAN BAG BOOGIE	Take 2 Bean Bags---throw them in rhythmic sequence. For example: Left – 2, right – 2, both -1. Continue at least 10 times.
4. EYE TO EYE	
5. JUMPING JACK FLASH	
6. JELLY ROLL	
7. CROSS WALK	
8. BALANCE BOARD BASH	While balancing, clap high 3 times above your head, then clap 3 times low behind your back, keep repeating while you count to 10.
9. CLIMB EVERY MOUNTAIN	
10. BEAM TEAM	Lock your hands together behind your head. Walk forward, then turn at midpoint on the beams.
11. MONSTER MASH	Stomp backwards!
12. PUPPY DOG CRAWL	
13. EYE CAN CONVERGE	
14. STRONG ARM PUSH	Push wall with **RIGHT** knee.
15. STEP BACK	

Minds-In-Motion WEEK 8

Each week changes will be made to some of the stations, increasing the skill level and intensity. If no change is designated, just continue with the basic movement as indicated on week 1:

1. SKIP TO MY LOU	
2. ELECTRIC SLIDE	
3. BEAN BAG BOOGIE	Hold 2 beanbags, one in each hand. Throw both into the air simultaneously and catch them when they come back down. Repeat 10 times.
4. EYE TO EYE	
5. JUMPING JACK FLASH	
6. JELLY ROLL	Roll with your arms held straight up, so you look like a straight pencil on the mat
7. CROSS WALK	
8. BALANCE BOARD BASH	While balancing, clap 2 times in front, then 2 times behind your back; keep repeating for a count of 10.
9. CLIMB EVERY MOUNTAIN	
10. BEAM TEAM	Hold both arms straight up in the air and walk down the beams, turning backwards at midpoint.
11. MONSTER MASH	
12. PUPPY DOG CRAWL	
13. EYE CAN CONVERGE	
14. STRONG ARM PUSH	Push wall with **LEFT** knee.
15. STEP BACK	

Minds-In-Motion WEEK 9

Each week changes will be made to some of the stations, increasing the skill level and intensity. If no change is designated, just continue with the basic movement as indicated on week 1:

1. SKIP TO MY LOU	
2. ELECTRIC SLIDE	
3. BEAN BAG BOOGIE	Throw 2 beanbags up in the air and catch them with opposite hands. Catch the bag thrown with the rt. hand in the left, and catch the bag thrown with the left in the right hand. Try it 10 times!
4. EYE TO EYE	
5. JUMPING JACK FLASH	
6. JELLY ROLL	Roll with your right arm held straight up by your ear while you roll; left arm down to your side.
7. CROSS WALK	
8. BALANCE BOARD BASH	While balancing, clap 3 times in front , then 3 times behind your back. Keep repeating for a count of 10.
9. CLIMB EVERY MOUNTAIN	
10. BEAM TEAM	Hold your hands locked behind you and elbows locked straight while walking down the beam, turning at midpoint.
11. MONSTER MASH	
12. PUPPY DOG CRAWL	
13. EYE CAN CONVERGE	
14. STRONG ARM PUSH	
15. STEP BACK	

Minds-In-Motion WEEK 10

Each week changes will be made to some of the stations, increasing the skill level and intensity. If no change is designated, just continue with the basic movement as indicated on week 1:

1. SKIP TO MY LOU	
2. ELECTRIC SLIDE	
3. BEAN BAG BOOGIE	Throw 1 beanbag up in the air and clap a rhythmic pattern (clap, clap, pause, clap) before catching it. Try it 10 times!
4. EYE TO EYE	Start counting while your eyes are being tracked.
5. JUMPING JACK FLASH	
6. JELLY ROLL	Roll with your left arm held straight up by your ear while you roll; right arm down to your side.
7. CROSS WALK	
8. BALANCE BOARD BASH	While balancing, clap 4 times in front, then 4 times behind your back. Keep repeating for a count of 10.
9. CLIMB EVERY MOUNTAIN	
10. BEAM TEAM	Hold your arms out in front of you. Hold your hands bent at the wrist, like a "stop" sign. Walk forward, then turn at midpoint.
11. MONSTER MASH	
12. PUPPY DOG CRAWL	Try to crawl backwards this week.
13. EYE CAN CONVERGE	
14. STRONG ARM PUSH	Push wall with just your fingertips!
15. STEP BACK	

Minds-In-Motion WEEK 11

Each week changes will be made to some of the stations, increasing the skill level and intensity. If no change is designated, just continue with the basic movement as indicated on week 1:

1. SKIP TO MY LOU	Hopscotch to a 2 feet, 1 foot, 2 feet, 1 foot, etc. pattern. (instead of skipping)
2. ELECTRIC SLIDE	
3. BEAN BAG BOOGIE	Throw 1 beanbag up in the air, clap your hands, slap your legs, before catching it. Try it 10 times.
4. EYE TO EYE	Start counting by tens while your eyes are being tracked.
5. JUMPING JACK FLASH	
6. JELLY ROLL	
7. CROSS WALK	
8. BALANCE BOARD BASH	Stand sideways, like you are surfing! [one foot in front of the other.] Try to keep your balance & count to 10.
9. CLIMB EVERY MOUNTAIN	
10. BEAM TEAM	Lock your fingers together straight out in front of you and walk backward down the whole beam.
11. MONSTER MASH	Stomp backward!
12. PUPPY DOG CRAWL	
13. EYE CAN CONVERGE	
14. STRONG ARM PUSH	Push wall with **RIGHT** elbow.
15. STEP BACK	

Minds-In-Motion WEEK 12

Each week changes will be made to some of the stations, increasing the skill level and intensity. If no change is designated, just continue with the basic movement as indicated on week 1:

1. SKIP TO MY LOU	Hopscotch to a 1-2-2 pattern. Hopscotch 1 foot, 2 feet, 2 feet; 1 foot, 2 feet, 2 feet, etc.
2. ELECTRIC SLIDE	
3. BEAN BAG BOOGIE	Throw 1 beanbag up in the air; turn around once, before catching it. Try it 10 times!
4. EYE TO EYE	Start counting by fives while your eyes are being tracked.
5. JUMPING JACK FLASH	
6. JELLY ROLL	Try to roll with your eyes closed.
7. CROSS WALK	Touch your feet BEHIND your back, touching right hand to left foot, etc. as you walk.
8. BALANCE BOARD BASH	Throw 1 beanbag up and catch it, while trying to balance. Repeat 10 times.
9. CLIMB EVERY MOUNTAIN	Climb over "mountain" backwards.
10. BEAM TEAM	Walk down the beam sideways leading with your right side.
11. MONSTER MASH	Stomp backward!
12. PUPPY DOG CRAWL	
13. EYE CAN CONVERGE	
14. STRONG ARM PUSH	Push wall with **LEFT** elbow.
15. STEP BACK	

Minds-In-Motion **WEEK 13**

Each week changes will be made to some of the stations, increasing the skill level and intensity. If no change is designated, just continue with the basic movement as indicated on week 1:

1. SKIP TO MY LOU	Hopscotch backwards! 1-2-1-2 pattern.
2. ELECTRIC SLIDE	
3. BEAN BAG BOOGIE	Throw 2 bean bags up in the air and clap 3 times before catching them.
4. EYE TO EYE	Start counting backwards from 30 while your eyes are being tracked. [You do not need to finish the count.]
5. JUMPING JACK FLASH	Increase jumping length by 6 inches.
6. JELLY ROLL	
7. CROSS WALK	Cross over and touch the bottom of your left shoe, then the bottom of your right shoe, then your left, etc. as you Crosswalk. Get your feet up high!
8. BALANCE BOARD BASH	As you balance, toss a bean bag back & forth level with your eyes.... 15 times.
9. CLIMB EVERY MOUNTAIN	
10. BEAM TEAM	Walk down the beam sideways leading with your left side.
11. MONSTER MASH	Stomp forward crossing over your right foot, then your left foot.
12. PUPPY DOG CRAWL	Crawl backwards this week.
13. EYE CAN CONVERGE	
14. STRONG ARM PUSH	Push with **BOTH** elbows!
15. STEP BACK	

Minds-In-Motion WEEK 14

Each week changes will be made to some of the stations, increasing the skill level and intensity. If no change is designated, just continue with the basic movement as indicated on week 1:

1. SKIP TO MY LOU	Skip with both arms pumping hard back and forth
2. ELECTRIC SLIDE	
3. BEAN BAG BOOGIE	Keep 2 bags in motion by throwing one up in the air, watching it reach the top of its trajectory, then throwing the other one up and so on for 10 times.
4. EYE TO EYE	Start counting backwards from 50 while your eyes are being tracked.
5. JUMPING JACK FLASH	
6. JELLY ROLL	Roll with your arms crossed in front of you.
7. CROSS WALK	Cross behind you and touch the bottom of your left shoe, then the bottom of your right shoe, then your left, etc. as you Crosswalk.
8. BALANCE BOARD BASH	As you balance, toss a bean bag back & forth level with your stomach.... 15 times.
9. CLIMB EVERY MOUNTAIN	
10. BEAM TEAM	Try to turn around in circles as you walk down the beam.
11. MONSTER MASH	Stomp forward crossing over your left then your right foot.
12. PUPPY DOG CRAWL	
13. EYE CAN CONVERGE	
14. STRONG ARM PUSH	Push with the back of your hands!
15. STEP BACK	

Minds-In-Motion **WEEK 15**

Each week changes will be made to some of the stations, increasing the skill level and intensity. If no change is designated, just continue with the basic movement as indicated on week 1:

1. SKIP TO MY LOU	RIGHT HAND BEHIND BACK
2. ELECTRIC SLIDE	RIGHT HAND BEHIND BACK
3. BEAN BAG BOOGIE	RIGHT HAND BEHIND BACK -Throw bag up with left hand, then turn hand over (upside down) to catch it.
4. EYE TO EYE	RIGHT HAND BEHIND BACK
5. JUMPING JACK FLASH	RIGHT HAND BEHIND BACK
6. JELLY ROLL	If it hurts to roll wtih your right hand behind back, please don't!
7. CROSS WALK	RIGHT HAND BEHIND BACK
8. BALANCE BOARD BASH	RIGHT HAND BEHIND BACK -Toss beanbag up & down with left hand while on board.
9. CLIMB EVERY MOUNTAIN	RIGHT HAND BEHIND BACK
10. BEAM TEAM	RIGHT HAND BEHIND BACK -Walk sideways on beam, turn at midpoint.
11. MONSTER MASH	RIGHT HAND BEHIND BACK
12. PUPPY DOG CRAWL	RIGHT HAND BEHIND BACK
13. EYE CAN CONVERGE	RIGHT HAND BEHIND BACK
14. STRONG ARM PUSH	RIGHT HAND BEHIND BACK
15. STEP BACK	RIGHT HAND BEHIND BACK

Minds-In-Motion WEEK 16

Each week changes will be made to some of the stations, increasing the skill level and intensity. If no change is designated, just continue with the basic movement as indicated on week 1:

1. SKIP TO MY LOU	LEFT HAND BEHIND BACK
2. ELECTRIC SLIDE	LEFT HAND BEHIND BACK
3. BEAN BAG BOOGIE	LEFT HAND BEHIND BACK -Throw bag up with right hand, then turn hand over (upside down) to catch it.
4. EYE TO EYE	LEFT HAND BEHIND BACK
5. JUMPING JACK FLASH	LEFT HAND BEHIND BACK
6. JELLY ROLL	If it hurts to put hand behind back, please don't!
7. CROSS WALK	LEFT HAND BEHIND BACK
8. BALANCE BOARD BASH	LEFT HAND BEHIND BACK -Toss beanbag up & catch ten times with right hand while on board.
9. CLIMB EVERY MOUNTAIN	LEFT HAND BEHIND BACK
10. BEAM TEAM	LEFT HAND BEHIND BACK -Walk sideways on beam, turn at midpoint.
11. MONSTER MASH	LEFT HAND BEHIND BACK
12. PUPPY DOG CRAWL	LEFT HAND BEHIND BACK
13. EYE CAN CONVERGE	LEFT HAND BEHIND BACK
14. STRONG ARM PUSH	LEFT HAND BEHIND BACK
15. STEP BACK	LEFT HAND BEHIND BACK

Minds-In-Motion WEEK 17

Each week changes will be made to some of the stations, increasing the skill level and intensity. If no change is designated, just continue with the basic movement as indicated on week 1:

1. SKIP TO MY LOU	HANDS ON TOP OF HEAD
2. ELECTRIC SLIDE	HANDS ON TOP OF HEAD
3. BEAN BAG BOOGIE	Take a beanbag in each hand and throw up into the air. Turn both hands over and upside down to catch one in the right hand and one in the left hand.
4. EYE TO EYE	Put hands on top of head while tracking with your eyes.
5. JUMPING JACK FLASH	HANDS ON TOP OF HEAD
6. JELLY ROLL	HANDS ON TOP OF HEAD
7. CROSS WALK	HANDS ON TOP OF HEAD
8. BALANCE BOARD BASH	HANDS ON TOP OF HEAD
9. CLIMB EVERY MOUNTAIN	HANDS ON TOP OF HEAD
10. BEAM TEAM	HANDS ON TOP OF HEAD [1ST beam forward; 2nd beam backward]
11. MONSTER MASH	Stomp backwards with hands on top of head
12. PUPPY DOG CRAWL	Crawl on knees with hands on top of head.
13. EYE CAN CONVERGE	HANDS ON TOP OF HEAD
14. STRONG ARM PUSH	Push with your back with hands on top of head.

Minds-In-Motion **WEEK 18**

Each week changes will be made to some of the stations, increasing the skill level and intensity. If no change is designated, just continue with the basic movement as indicated on week 1:

1. SKIP TO MY LOU	Take giant steps <u>sliding</u> right foot, then left foot (like you are ice skating) leaning forward and swinging arms side to side.
2. ELECTRIC SLIDE	
3. BEAN BAG BOOGIE	While hopping on right foot, throw a beanbag up in the air with left hand and catch it when it comes down. Do this 10 times.
4. EYE TO EYE	Say [not sing] the alphabet while your eyes are tracking.
5. JUMPING JACK FLASH	
6. JELLY ROLL	Roll with your legs crossed at ankles.
7. CROSS WALK	
8. BALANCE BOARD BASH	Toss a beanbag from rt. hand to left [over the rainbow] back & forth for 10 times.
9. CLIMB EVERY MOUNTAIN	
10. BEAM TEAM	Hold a beanbag under your chin while walking forward, then reverse & walk backwards at midpoint.
11. MONSTER MASH	
12. PUPPY DOG CRAWL	Crawl on knees with hands behind back.
13. EYE CAN CONVERGE	
14. STRONG ARM PUSH	Push with your **RIGHT** shoulder.
15. STEP BACK	

Minds-In-Motion WEEK 19

Each week changes will be made to some of the stations, increasing the skill level and intensity. If no change is designated, just continue with the basic movement as indicated on week 1:

1. SKIP TO MY LOU	Take giant steps <u>leaping</u> from right foot to left foot (almost like ice skating) leaning forward and swinging arms side to side.
2. ELECTRIC SLIDE	
3. BEAN BAG BOOGIE	While hopping on your left foot, throw a beanbag up in the air with your right hand and catch it when it comes down. Do this 10 times.
4. EYE TO EYE	Say the days of the week while your eyes are tracking
5. JUMPING JACK FLASH	
6. JELLY ROLL	
7. CROSS WALK	
8. BALANCE BOARD BASH	Balance standing sideways on the board. Count backwards from 20. (from 10 for K & 1st graders)
9. CLIMB EVERY MOUNTAIN	
10. BEAM TEAM	Carry a beanbag on top of your head while walking forward, then turn backwards at midpoint.
11. MONSTER MASH	
12. PUPPY DOG CRAWL	Crawl on knees with arms folded across chest.
13. EYE CAN CONVERGE	
14. STRONG ARM PUSH	Push with your left shoulder
15. STEP BACK	

Minds-In-Motion WEEK 20

Each week changes will be made to some of the stations, increasing the skill level and intensity. If no change is designated, just continue with the basic movement as indicated on week 1:

1. SKIP TO MY LOU	Hopscotch to the pattern of: 1 – 1 – 2 – 2
2. ELECTRIC SLIDE	
3. BEAN BAG BOOGIE	While hopping on both feet, throw a beanbag up in the air and catch it with both hands when it comes down.
4. EYE TO EYE	Say the days of the week backwards while your eyes are tracking.
5. JUMPING JACK FLASH	
6. JELLY ROLL	
7. CROSS WALK	
8. BALANCE BOARD BASH	Balance standing sideways [facing opposite side from last week] on the board. Count backwards from 20 (count from 10 for K).
9. CLIMB EVERY MOUNTAIN	
10. BEAM TEAM	Carry 2 beanbags stacked on top of your head while walking forward, then turn backwards at midpoint.
11. MONSTER MASH	Take scissor-steps as you stomp behind you to the back [right foot stomps on left pad, then left foot stomps on right pad, etc]
12. PUPPY DOG CRAWL	Army crawl on tummy.
13. EYE CAN CONVERGE	
14. STRONG ARM PUSH	Push with both shoulders to the front
15. STEP BACK	

Minds-In-Motion WEEK 21

Each week changes will be made to some of the stations, increasing the skill level and intensity. If no change is designated, just continue with the basic movement as indicated on week 1:

1. SKIP TO MY LOU	Hopscotch to the pattern of : R – L – 2 – 2 (one foot R – one foot L – 2 feet – 2 feet
2. ELECTRIC SLIDE	
3. BEAN BAG BOOGIE	Hop on both feet while twirling around, throw bean bag up and catch with both hands- 10 times. Easter bunny practice!!
4. EYE TO EYE	Say the months of the year while your eyes are tracking
5. JUMPING JACK FLASH	Add another tape line of a different color 6-12 inches further: encourage students to jump farther!
6. JELLY ROLL	
7. CROSS WALK	Cross arms over chest and touch elbows to knees as you Cross Walk.
8. BALANCE BOARD BASH	
9. CLIMB EVERY MOUNTAIN	
10. BEAM TEAM	Carry 2 beanbags on top of your head while walking sideways down beam, turning at midpoint.
11. MONSTER MASH	Hold hands on top of your head; take scissor-steps as you stomp behind you to the back [right foot stomps on left pad, then left foot stomps on right pad, etc]
12. PUPPY DOG CRAWL	Army crawl on tummy, making sure opposite arm and leg are moving at same time.
13. EYE CAN CONVERGE	
14. STRONG ARM PUSH	Push with both shoulders to the back.
15. STEP BACK	

Minds-In-Motion WEEK 22

Each week changes will be made to some of the stations, increasing the skill level and intensity. If no change is designated, just continue with the basic movement as indicated on week 1:

1. SKIP TO MY LOU	Balance a bean bag on top of head throughout the whole maze!
2. ELECTRIC SLIDE	Balance a bean bag on top of head throughout the whole maze!
3. BEAN BAG BOOGIE	Pick up another beanbag and toss it from hand to hand (while carrying beanbag on your head)
4. EYE TO EYE	Balance a bean bag on top of head throughout the whole maze!
5. JUMPING JACK FLASH	Balance a bean bag on top of head throughout the whole maze!
6. JELLY ROLL	[hold bean bag on head for this one!]
7. CROSS WALK	Balance a bean bag on top of head throughout the whole maze!
8. BALANCE BOARD BASH	Balance a bean bag on top of head throughout the whole maze!
9. CLIMB EVERY MOUNTAIN	Balance a bean bag on top of head throughout the whole maze!
10. BEAM TEAM	Balance a bean bag on top of head throughout the whole maze!
11. MONSTER MASH	Balance a bean bag on top of head throughout the whole maze!
12. PUPPY DOG CRAWL	Army crawl with beanbag laying on back.
13. EYE CAN CONVERGE	Balance a bean bag on top of head throughout the whole maze!
14. STRONG ARM PUSH	Balance a bean bag on top of head throughout the whole maze!
15. STEP BACK	Balance a bean bag on top of head throughout the whole maze!

Minds-In-Motion **WEEK 23**

Each week changes will be made to some of the stations, increasing the skill level and intensity. If no change is designated, just continue with the basic movement as indicated on week 1:

1. SKIP TO MY LOU	Balance a beanbag on your right shoulder to carry throughout the whole maze!
2. ELECTRIC SLIDE	Balance a beanbag on your right shoulder to carry throughout the whole maze!
3. BEAN BAG BOOGIE	Take your beanbag in your hands and throw it into the air. Then try to hit it with your right shoulder (using your shoulder as a "bat") and catch it back in your hands. Try this 10 times. Good luck...it is hard!!
4. EYE TO EYE	Balance a beanbag on your right shoulder to carry throughout the whole maze!
5. JUMPING JACK FLASH	Balance a beanbag on your right shoulder even while jumping.
6. JELLY ROLL	[Hold it on your right shoulder while you roll!]
7. CROSS WALK	Balance a beanbag on your right shoulder to carry throughout the whole maze!
8. BALANCE BOARD BASH	Balance a beanbag on your right shoulder to carry throughout the whole maze!
9. CLIMB EVERY MOUNTAIN	Balance a beanbag on your right shoulder to carry throughout the whole maze!
10. BEAM TEAM	Balance a beanbag on your right shoulder to carry throughout the whole maze!
11. MONSTER MASH	Be sure to stomp backwards this week with bean bag on right shoulder.
12. PUPPY DOG CRAWL	Army crawl with beanbag on right shoulder.
13. EYE CAN CONVERGE	Balance a beanbag on your right shoulder to carry throughout the whole maze!
14. STRONG ARM PUSH	Push with both hands while carrying the beanbag on your right shoulder.
15. STEP BACK	Balance a beanbag on your right shoulder to carry throughout the whole maze!

Minds-In-Motion WEEK 24

Each week changes will be made to some of the stations, increasing the skill level and intensity. If no change is designated, just continue with the basic movement as indicated on week 1:

1. SKIP TO MY LOU	Balance a beanbag on your left shoulder to carry throughout the whole maze!
2. ELECTRIC SLIDE	Balance a beanbag on your left shoulder to carry throughout the whole maze!
3. BEAN BAG BOOGIE	Take your beanbag in your hands and throw it into the air. Then try to hit it with your left shoulder (using your shoulder as a "bat") and catch it back in your hands. Try this 10 times. Good luck...it is hard!!
4. EYE TO EYE	Balance a beanbag on your left shoulder to carry throughout the whole maze!
5. JUMPING JACK FLASH	Balance a beanbag on left shoulder even while jumping.
6. JELLY ROLL	(Hold it on your left shoulder while you roll)
7. CROSS WALK	Balance a beanbag on your left shoulder to carry throughout the whole maze!
8. BALANCE BOARD BASH	Balance a beanbag on your left shoulder to carry throughout the whole maze!
9. CLIMB EVERY MOUNTAIN	Balance a beanbag on your left shoulder to carry throughout the whole maze!
10. BEAM TEAM	Balance a beanbag on your left shoulder to carry throughout the whole maze!
11. MONSTER MASH	Be sure to stomp backwards again this week with beanbag on left shoulder.
12. PUPPY DOG CRAWL	Army crawl with beanbag on left shoulder.
13. EYE CAN CONVERGE	Balance a beanbag on your left shoulder to carry throughout the whole maze!
14. STRONG ARM PUSH	Push with both hands while carrying the beanbag on your left shoulder.
15. STEP BACK	Balance a beanbag on your left shoulder to carry throughout the whole maze!

Minds-In-Motion WEEK 25

Each week changes will be made to some of the stations, increasing the skill level and intensity. If no change is designated, just continue with the basic movement as indicated on week 1:

1. SKIP TO MY LOU	Pick up 2 beanbags - putting one on each shoulder to carry throughout the whole maze! Try not to hold onto beanbags as you skip!
2. ELECTRIC SLIDE	Carry them on your shoulders while you slide.
3. BEAN BAG BOOGIE	Pick up another beanbag and toss it from hand to hand (while carrying a beanbag on both of your shoulders.)
4. EYE TO EYE	Carry beanbags on shoulders while having eyes tracked.
5. JUMPING JACK FLASH	Increase jump length tape lines by 6 inches. Try not to hold onto bean bags as you jump!
6. JELLY ROLL	Hold them on your shoulders while you roll.
7. CROSS WALK	Carry them on your shoulders while you crosswalk.
8. BALANCE BOARD BASH	Carry them on your shoulders while you balance.
9. CLIMB EVERY MOUNTAIN	Carry them on your shoulders while you step over.
10. BEAM TEAM	Carry them on your shoulders while you walk on beams.
11. MONSTER MASH	Carry them on your shoulders while you stomp.
12. PUPPY DOG CRAWL	Carry them on your back while you crawl.
13. EYE CAN CONVERGE	Carry them on your shoulders while you converge your eyes.
14. STRONG ARM PUSH	Carry them on your shoulders while you push.
15. STEP BACK	Carry them on your shoulders while you step back.

Minds-In-Motion WEEK 26

Each week changes will be made to some of the stations, increasing the skill level and intensity. If no change is designated, just continue with the basic movement as indicated on week 1:

1. SKIP TO MY LOU	Go through the whole maze on your tiptoes! Skip on your tiptoes!
2. ELECTRIC SLIDE	On your tiptoes!
3. BEAN BAG BOOGIE	Throw a bean bag up and hit it with your head, then try to catch it while walking on your tiptoes.
4. EYE TO EYE	While tracking, name everything you can think of that is pointed. Keep on your tiptoes!
5. JUMPING JACK FLASH	Jump on your tiptoes!
6. JELLY ROLL	Point your toes while you roll!
7. CROSS WALK	Cross walk on your tiptoes!
8. BALANCE BOARD BASH	Have a beanbag placed on each balance board. Throw a beanbag up and try to catch it while balancing on your toes. Repeat 10 times.
9. CLIMB EVERY MOUNTAIN	On tiptoes!
10. BEAM TEAM	On tiptoes!
11. MONSTER MASH	On tiptoes!
12. PUPPY DOG CRAWL	Crawl with hands on floor with your feet up on tiptoes.
13. EYE CAN CONVERGE	On tiptoes!
14. STRONG ARM PUSH	On tiptoes!
15. STEP BACK	On tiptoes!

Each week changes will be made to some of the stations, increasing the skill level and intensity. If no change is designated, just continue with the basic movement as indicated on week 1:

1. SKIP TO MY LOU	
2. ELECTRIC SLIDE	Clap your hands in a rhythmic pattern as you Electric Slide.
3. BEAN BAG BOOGIE	Throw a bean bag up and hit it with your right knee, then try to catch it. Continue ten times.
4. EYE TO EYE	While tracking, name everything you can think of that is green.
5. JUMPING JACK FLASH	
6. JELLY ROLL	Roll with your right arm held straight up by your ear, left arm down by your side.
7. CROSS WALK	Cross over and touch your left foot, then your right foot, then your left, etc. as you Crosswalk. Get your feet up high!
8. BALANCE BOARD BASH	Have a beanbag on each balance board. As you balance, throw the beanbag up in the air, clap your hands, catch the beanbag.
9. CLIMB EVERY MOUNTAIN	Change the mountain to climb over! Use boxes, steps, building blocks, etc.
10. BEAM TEAM	Clap your hands as you walk down the beam. Clap your hands and keep a rhythmn. Needed next week: 12 canned foods - all sizes
11. MONSTER MASH	
12. PUPPY DOG CRAWL	
13. EYE CAN CONVERGE	
14. STRONG ARM PUSH	Push with the right side of your body against the wall.
15. STEP BACK	

Minds-In-Motion WEEK 28

Each week changes will be made to some of the stations, increasing the skill level and intensity. If no change is designated, just continue with the basic movement as indicated on week 1:

1. SKIP TO MY LOU	Try skipping in circular movements.
2. ELECTRIC SLIDE	
3. BEAN BAG BOOGIE	Throw a bean bag up and hit it with your left knee, then try to catch it. Continue ten times.
4. EYE TO EYE	Name all the nouns (persons, places or things) you can think of while your eyes are tracked.
5. JUMPING JACK FLASH	
6. JELLY ROLL	Roll with your left arm held straight up by your ear, right arm down by your side.
7. CROSS WALK	Cross over and touch your left foot with your right index finger, then your right foot with left index finger, etc. as you crosswalk.
8. BALANCE BOARD BASH	Try to balance with your eyes closed!
9. CLIMB EVERY MOUNTAIN	
10. BEAM TEAM	(Place a container full of unbreakable canned goods at beginning of Beam Team.) Pick up a can as you walk sideways down the beam. Hold it straight out in front of you in both hands. Lay can of food in another container at end of beams.
11. MONSTER MASH	Hop on each pad with both feet.
12. PUPPY DOG CRAWL	Army crawl under rods in cones (or any other structure you have to crawl under)
13. EYE CAN CONVERGE	
14. STRONG ARM PUSH	Push with the left side of your body against the wall.
15. STEP BACK	

Minds-In-Motion **WEEK 29**

Each week changes will be made to some of the stations, increasing the skill level and intensity. If no change is designated, just continue with the basic movement as indicated on week 1:

1. SKIP TO MY LOU	Try to skip sideways leading with your right side!!
2. ELECTRIC SLIDE	
3. BEAN BAG BOOGIE	Throw the beanbag up with your right hand, hit it with your left wrist, then catch it with your right hand. Continue 10 times.
4. EYE TO EYE	Name colors while your eyes are being tracked.
5. JUMPING JACK FLASH	
6. JELLY ROLL	
7. CROSS WALK	Cross behind your body and touch the bottom of your left shoe, then the bottom or your right shoe, then your left, etc. as you crosswalk.
8. BALANCE BOARD BASH	As you balance, toss a bean bag back and forth level with your stomach as fast as you can... 15 times.
9. CLIMB EVERY MOUNTAIN	
10. BEAM TEAM	Hold a can in your right hand out straight to the side as you walk down the beam.
11. MONSTER MASH	Stomp scissors-step backwards. Cross one foot behind the other and really stomp!
12. PUPPY DOG CRAWL	Army crawl on tummy.
13. EYE CAN CONVERGE	
14. STRONG ARM PUSH	Make fists and push against wall with fists.
15. STEP BACK	

Minds-In-Motion WEEK 30

Each week changes will be made to some of the stations, increasing the skill level and intensity. If no change is designated, just continue with the basic movement as indicated on week 1:

1. SKIP TO MY LOU	Try to skip sideways leading with your left side!!
2. ELECTRIC SLIDE	
3. BEAN BAG BOOGIE	Throw the beanbag up with your left hand, hit it with your right wrist, then catch it with your left hand. Continue 10 times.
4. EYE TO EYE	Recite your favorite foods while your eyes are being tracked.
5. JUMPING JACK FLASH	JUMP BACKWARDS.
6. JELLY ROLL	
7. CROSS WALK	Cross behind and touch the bottom of your left shoe, then the bottom or your right shoe, then your left, etc. as you crosswalk.
8. BALANCE BOARD BASH	As you balance, toss a bean bag back and forth level with your neck as fast as you can... 15 times. Follow it with your nose.
9. CLIMB EVERY MOUNTAIN	
10. BEAM TEAM	Hold a can with your left hand out straight to the side as you walk down the beam. Try to hold it upright on your palm.
11. MONSTER MASH	Hop backwards on each stomping pad.
12. PUPPY DOG CRAWL	Puppy Crawl BACKWARDS.
13. EYE CAN CONVERGE	
14. STRONG ARM PUSH	Push with your right knee on the wall.
15. STEP BACK	

Minds-In-Motion WEEK 31

Each week changes will be made to some of the stations, increasing the skill level and intensity. If no change is designated, just continue with the basic movement as indicated on week 1:

1. SKIP TO MY LOU	Try to skip backward!!
2. ELECTRIC SLIDE	
3. BEAN BAG BOOGIE	Throw the beanbag up and hit it with your right knee; catch it. Hit it with your left knee; catch it. Continue 10 times.
4. EYE TO EYE	Recite your favorite colors while your eyes are being tracked.
5. JUMPING JACK FLASH	
6. JELLY ROLL	
7. CROSS WALK	Cross over and touch the bottom of your left shoe, then the bottom or your right shoe, then your left, etc. as you crosswalk.
8. BALANCE BOARD BASH	As you balance, toss a bean bag back and forth level with your eyes as fast as you can... 15 times.
9. CLIMB EVERY MOUNTAIN	Walk over the obstacle backwards.
10. BEAM TEAM	Pick up a can and carry it over your head as you walk down the beam.
11. MONSTER MASH	Interlock legs and jump on each stomping pad.
12. PUPPY DOG CRAWL	ARMY CRAWL BACKWARDS.
13. EYE CAN CONVERGE	
14. STRONG ARM PUSH	Push with your left knee against the wall.
15. STEP BACK	

Minds-In-Motion **WEEK 32**

Each week changes will be made to some of the stations, increasing the skill level and intensity. If no change is designated, just continue with the basic movement as indicated on week 1:

1. SKIP TO MY LOU	Practice skipping backward again!!
2. ELECTRIC SLIDE	
3. BEAN BAG BOOGIE	Throw the beanbag up in the air, spin around and try to catch it.
4. EYE TO EYE	Name all the farm animals you can while eyes are being tracked.
5. JUMPING JACK FLASH	Jump backwards.
6. JELLY ROLL	
7. CROSS WALK	Cross walk with your legs out straight in front of you. Touch your opposite knee as your leg comes up straight.
8. BALANCE BOARD BASH	As you balance, toss a bean bag back and forth with your hands above your head.
9. CLIMB EVERY MOUNTAIN	
10. BEAM TEAM	Hold a can with both hands behind your back while you walk down the beam.
11. MONSTER MASH	Do the twist while stomping forward.
12. PUPPY DOG CRAWL	Crawl backward on your knees, with hands on hips.
13. EYE CAN CONVERGE	
14. STRONG ARM PUSH	Invent a new way to push the wall!
15. STEP BACK	

Minds-In-Motion WEEK 33

Each week changes will be made to some of the stations, increasing the skill level and intensity. If no change is designated, just continue with the basic movement as indicated on week 1:

1. SKIP TO MY LOU	Skip forward while throwing and catching a bean bag with both hands!!
2. ELECTRIC SLIDE	
3. BEAN BAG BOOGIE	Throw the beanbag up in the air, bend down and touch the ground, then stand up and try to catch it.
4. EYE TO EYE	Name as many flavors of ice cream as you can while eyes are being tracked.
5. JUMPING JACK FLASH	Jump backward.
6. JELLY ROLL	
7. CROSS WALK	Cross walk with your legs out straight in front of you. Touch your opposite mid-calf as your leg comes up straight.
8. BALANCE BOARD BASH	As you balance, toss a bean bag back and forth at knee level, as fast as you can.
9. CLIMB EVERY MOUNTAIN	
10. BEAM TEAM	Hold a can straight out in front of you with both hands while you walk down the beam.
11. MONSTER MASH	Do the twist while stomping backward!!
12. PUPPY DOG CRAWL	Crawl backward on your knees, with arms held straight up in the air.
13. EYE CAN CONVERGE	
14. STRONG ARM PUSH	
15. STEP BACK	

Minds-In-Motion WEEK 34

Each week changes will be made to some of the stations, increasing the skill level and intensity. If no change is designated, just continue with the basic movement as indicated on week 1:

1. SKIP TO MY LOU	Skip forward while tossing and catching a bean bag in your right hand.
2. ELECTRIC SLIDE	
3. BEAN BAG BOOGIE	Throw the beanbag up in the air, bend down and touch the ground with both hands and then stand and try to catch it.
4. EYE TO EYE	Name as many cars as you can while eyes are being tracked.
5. JUMPING JACK FLASH	Jump backward with eyes closed.
6. JELLY ROLL	Roll as fast as you can!
7. CROSS WALK	Cross walk with your legs out straight in front of you. Try to touch your opposite toe as your leg comes up straight.
8. BALANCE BOARD BASH	As you balance, toss a bean bag around and around your waist as fast as you can.
9. CLIMB EVERY MOUNTAIN	Roll as fast as you can!
10. BEAM TEAM	Hold a can straight out in front of your stomach with both hands while you walk down the beam.
11. MONSTER MASH	Do the WAVE while stomping backward!!
12. PUPPY DOG CRAWL	Try to crawl SIDEWAYS on your knees.
13. EYE CAN CONVERGE	
14. STRONG ARM PUSH	Invent another way to push the wall.
15. STEP BACK	

Minds-In-Motion WEEK 35

Each week changes will be made to some of the stations, increasing the skill level and intensity. If no change is designated, just continue with the basic movement as indicated on week 1:

1. SKIP TO MY LOU	Skip forward while tossing and catching a bean bag in your left hand.
2. ELECTRIC SLIDE	
3. BEAN BAG BOOGIE	Throw the beanbag up in the air, make a hoop with your arms forming a circle, then have beanbag make a basket through the hoop.
4. EYE TO EYE	Name as many boys' names as you can while eyes are being tracked.
5. JUMPING JACK FLASH	Jump on your right foot only.
6. JELLY ROLL	
7. CROSS WALK	Cross walk and touch your elbows to your knees.
8. BALANCE BOARD BASH	As you balance, toss a bean bag around and around your head as fast as you can.
9. CLIMB EVERY MOUNTAIN	
10. BEAM TEAM	Try to walk in circles as you go down the beams with a can held in your hands.
11. MONSTER MASH	Stomp on your heels.
12. PUPPY DOG CRAWL	Crawl sideways on your knees leading with your right side.
13. EYE CAN CONVERGE	
14. STRONG ARM PUSH	
15. STEP BACK	

Minds-In-Motion WEEK 36

Each week changes will be made to some of the stations, increasing the skill level and intensity. If no change is designated, just continue with the basic movement as indicated on week 1:

1. SKIP TO MY LOU	Skip forward while tossing and catching a bean bag from left hand to right hand.
2. ELECTRIC SLIDE	While sliding, swing your arms back and forth.
3. BEAN BAG BOOGIE	Throw the beanbag up in the air with your left hand. make a hoop with your right arm forming a circle then have the beanbag make a basket through your hoop.
4. EYE TO EYE	Name as many girls' names as you can while eyes are being tracked.
5. JUMPING JACK FLASH	Jump on your left foot only.
6. JELLY ROLL	Cross your arms keeping your legs straight as you roll.
7. CROSS WALK	
8. BALANCE BOARD BASH	As you balance, pass bean bag in a figure 8 around and in between your knees as fast as you can.
9. CLIMB EVERY MOUNTAIN	
10. BEAM TEAM	Try to walk in circles as you go down the beams with a can held under your right arm pit.
11. MONSTER MASH	Stomp on your heels.
12. PUPPY DOG CRAWL	Crawl sideways on your knees leading with your left side.
13. EYE CAN CONVERGE	
14. STRONG ARM PUSH	Cross your arms, making an X, then push with both hands.
15. STEP BACK	Step back without holding on to the railing.

> *"Vision is the dominant human sense, the most complicated and far more significant than either speech or hearing in most learning situations."* —*Dr. James Kimple, 1997*

SUGGESTED WEBSITES:

www.Bal-a-vis-x.com—Balance-auditory-visual exercises

www.autoskill.com—Academy of Reading and Math

www.pavevision.org—Parents Active for Vision Education

www.balametrics.com—Dr.Belgau's website

www.MiMlearning.com—The Minds-in-Motion website!

Obstacles that Face the 21st Century Learner

- Can't pay attention; easily distracted
- Acts out socially
- Frequent melt-downs
- Tends to whine a lot
- Talks too loud
- Covers ears when loud sounds
- Gets in others' personal space
- Frustrated at school or at home
- Toe walker or quite clumsy
- Scared to try new things
- Hyper!! Can't stop moving or very slow moving
- Hard to make transitions
- Hard time keeping hands to oneself

Bibliography

AYRES, JEAN. Sensory Integration and the Child, Understanding Hidden Sensory Challenges, 25th Anniversary Edition. Los Angeles, CA: Western Psychological Services, 2005.

BARRY, SUSAN. Fixing my Gaze. Philadelphia, PA: Perseus Books, 2009.

BELGAU, FRANK, AND BEVERLEY BELGAU. A Perceptual Motor and Visual Perception Handbook of Developmental Activities for Schools, Clinics, Parents, and Preschool Programs. Balametrics. Port Washington, WA, 2000.

BLOMBERG, HARALD. Movements That Heal. Australia: Book Pal, 2011.

CHEATUM, BILLYE ANN. Physical Activities for Improving Children's Learning and Behavior, A Guide to Sensory Motor Development. Human Kinetics, 2000.

DELACATO, CARL. A New Start for the Child with Reading Problems: A Manual for Parents, Revised and Updated Edition. Morton, PA: Morton Books, 1982.

DENNISON, PAUL E. BRAIN GYM: Simple Activities for Whole Brain Integration. Ventura, CA: Edu-Kinesthetics, Inc., 1986.

---BRAIN GYM, Teacher's Edition, Revised. Ventura, CA: Edu-Kinesthetics, Inc., 1994.

DOIDGE, NORMAN. The Brain that Changes Itself. New York: Penguin Books, 2007.

DOMAN, GLENN. How to Teach your Baby to be Physically Suburb. Philadelphia, PA: The Better Baby Press, 1991.

GODDARD, SALLY. Reflexes, Learning and Behavior, A Window into the Child's Mind. Eugene, OR: Fern Ridge Press, 2002.

---. The Well Balanced Child, United Kingdom: Hawthorn Press, 2004.

GOLD, SVEA. If Kids Just Came with Instruction Sheets!, Eugene, OR: Fern Ridge Press, 1997.

GREEN, NANCY SOKOL. Adventure Trails. Brain Highways, 2003.

HANNAFORD, CARLA. Smart Moves: Why Learning Is Not All In Your Head. Arlington, VA: Great Ocean Publishers, 1995.

---. The Dominance Factor: How Knowing Your Dominant Eye, Ear, Hand and Foot Can Improve Your Learning. Arlington, VA: Great Ocean Publishers, 1997.

HUBERT, BILL. Bal-A-Vis-X: Rhythmic/Balance/Auditory/Vision Exercises for Brain and Brain/Body Integration. Wichita, KS: Bal-A-Vis-X, Inc., 2001.

KIMPLE, JAMES. Eye Q and the Efficient Learner. Optometric Extension Program, 1997.

KRANOWITZ, CAROL S. Answers to Questions Teachers Ask about Sensory Integration. Las Vegas, NV: Sensory Resources, 2003.

---. The Out of Sync Child: Recognizing and Coping With Sensory Integration Dysfunction. New York: Skylight Press, 1998.

LEVINSON, HAROLD. Phobia Free. New York: Evans & Co., Inc. 1986

LEVINSON, HAROLD. Smart But Feeling Dumb. New York: Warner Books, 1994.

LOUV, RICHARD. Last Child in the Woods. Chapel Hill, N.C.: Algonquin Books, 2008.

MCCREDIE, SCOTT. Balance: In Search of the Lost Sense. New York: Little, Brown & Co., 2007.

MEDINA, JOHN. Brain Rules. Seattle, WA: Pear Press, 2008.

O'DELL, NANCY, PHD. AND PATRICIA COOK. Stopping Hyperactivity – A New Solution. Garden City Park, NY: Avery Publishing Group, 1997.

QUIRK, NORMA. The Relationship of Learning Problems and Classroom Performance to Sensory Integration. 1990.

RATEY, JOHN. Spark: The Revolutionary New Science of Exercise and the Brain. New York: Little, Brown. and Co., 2008.

Success stories

A FIRST GRADE TEACHER, who runs a Minds-in-Motion Maze and has been implementing it for almost 4 years, writes:

Hannah is the little girl that has a 1 inch thick IEP. Most of it is "physical therapy" kinds of issues. You can see that her handwriting as well as her sentence formation has drastically improved! Her PT now only has her on consult. She also tested out of speech therapy. The PT was just amazed at the progress Hannah has made in such a short time!

Larry is a boy who came in January and was not on grade level in reading. He needed to test into a level 5 and he was only at level 2 and his word list was at 0. In just about a month and a half he managed to make it onto grade level and he moved 9 levels on his word list. He topped out! There are only 9 levels in all. He is so much happier. He participates a lot now!

There was another boy that moved here in late December. His old principal called us and warned us about him. He said that he was absolutely one of the worst kids he had ever dealt with. He said he was mean and uncontrollable and that he was extremely low academically. In fact, he was labeled mildly autistic. I was really worried! When he finally came to me, he wasn't using much speech and he was on about a Pre-Kindergarten level. He was also unable to do any part of the Minds-in-Motion Maze. After about 1 week he was doing all parts with some help. Then eventually, he could do the Maze completely by himself. He was participating sooooo much in class that it was hard for others to get a comment in. I really enjoyed him. He turned out to be the sweetest child in the class--not the least bit of a behavior problem! He was also NOT AUTISTIC! He was really a joy!
--KV

I am an occupational therapist for some county schools in Indiana. We have the Maze set up in several of our schools and have seen great results so far and have been glad to have a resource like the maze to tap into and give to our teachers as a resource. We get many questions about the maze and your program from our parents and others in the community. We often direct people to your website. Thank you for your time and assistance!
--BS, MS, OTR

FROM PRINCIPAL, M. MCDONOUGH, College Corner Union Elementary, Ohio:

I'll start with a fabulous example...Last Friday, we staged a full blown lockdown and evacuation drill. Picture this: The entire school exiting the front doors and walking down the block to a local church, walking into the pews, taking their ID cards, and sitting quietly waiting for further directions. Each and every student walked single file, straight line, hands to themselves... no running, pushing ahead, falling, spinning, talking, etc...all the usual things you would expect to see with a mass exodus....well we, here at CCUS, turned to each other and stated a simple 3 word phrase (that has become a habit around here), "Minds-*in-Motion*!" Truly, the town crime watch committee even commented on the incredible organization and self-control that each child displayed!!! WOW!! That would not have been the case 3 years ago!!!!

AND, we see stories like that every day...the number of discipline referrals to my office has dropped to nearly non-existent. If kiddos DO show up in my office...they usually have to take a MIM break...with me! Students have learned to take, 'mind minutes' for themselves.

The halls are filled with orderly skipping, dancing, moving in some way or another...and ways that students have themselves invented. We have added math facts, number counting (by 2's, 3's etc), abc's and any number of academic necessities to our movements.

This morning, we hosted a Cincinnati school to talk to them about our reading program...well, as usual, we credited Minds-in-Motion for the incredible amount of self-directedness that these folks observed in our students.

And, student engagement has soared since we implemented MIM...and we keep raising the bar with it!! It is serious business around here...no messing around with MIM... because we get serious RESULTS!!

Here is a beginning list of our qualitative data
- Self-control
- Better handwriting
- Increased fluency in reading and writing
- Better organization—students and adults!
- Increased self-esteem/better behavior/less discipline referrals
- Cerebral Palsy students being released sooner from OT
- Decreased identification of spec. ed. students

About the Author

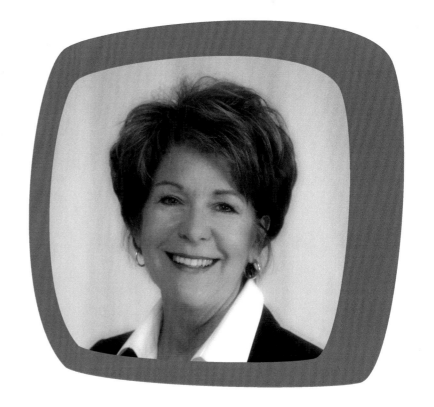

CANDACE S. MEYER, M.S., the founder and developer of Minds-in-Motion, Inc. a unique advanced development program, has over 30 years experience in the field of education. Graduating Summa Cum Laude with a Master's endorsement in Corrective Reading, she has worked her way through the educational world, from teaching grades K – 4, being a writing specialist in grades K-5, training staff in professional development, to being the reading specialist for a county school district in Indiana, and Title I Federal Program Coordinator for ten of those years. Drawing upon this hands-on experience, Meyer has spent the last decade personally researching the correlation between vestibular development and learning difficulties while developing her groundbreaking Minds-in-Motion program. Using a clinical device originally invented for NASA by Dr. Lew Nashner to measure the prolonged effects of weightlessness on the vestibular functionality of astronauts, Meyer has been conducting assessments, collecting SBR (Scientifically Based Research) data, and developing personalized improvement plans for students with great success.

To date she has collected data on 1300+ students, ranging from gifted PhD college students to struggling country, inner city, and rural mountain children. The comparative, clinical data shows that when students, of any age or race or socio-economic level, have opportunities to build strong neurological foundations by activating sensory-motor integration processes, they become positioned to learn with ease and success, and are able to reach a higher potential. Meyer owns two state-of-the-art Minds-in-Motion Centers in Louisville, KY and Carmel, IN. She has personally trained over 800 teachers in ten states on her Minds-in-Motion Maze program.

Notes

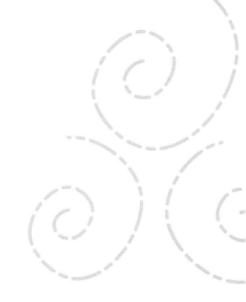